Senior Stick Fit

Senior Exercise Program

By

Sensei James Birkle

Senior Stick Fit

Senior Exercise Program

By Sensei Jim Birkle

This publication is designed to provide accurate and authoritative information in regard to the subject matter covered. It is sold the understanding that the publisher is not engaged in rendering legal, accounting, or other professional services. If legal advice or other expert assistance is required, the services of a competent professional person should be sought

First Published, 2014

Second Reprint, 2015

Printed in the United States of America

Thank You For Buying This Book

I was hoping you could help your fellow book enthusiasts out and when you have a free second leave your honest feedback about this book. I certainly want to thank you in advance for doing this.

ACKNOWLEDGEMENTS

A manual of this sort can never be considered the sole creation of one person. There are several people who assisted and supported me in this endeavor in one way or another. I would like to take this opportunity to mention their names and thank them for their assistance.

Professor Ernie Boggs

Professor Boggs a co-founder of *"Stick Fit"* has been inducted into multiple Martial Arts Hall of Fames and one of only five Americans ever to be inducted into the Pantheon Hall of Sports in Geneva, Switzerland. Mr. Boggs is a former middleweight world champion and the very first American to ever win a world title in jujitsu. He has also competed on the national and international circuit, excelling in traditional karate and professional kickboxing as well. - Mr. Boggs has 46 years of in depth martial arts training, largely under the guidance of legendary masters as well as some of the world's leading weapons and self-defense elite. He has achieved expert level in many combat systems including 5th degree black belt in karate and 7th degree in jujitsu. He is considered one of the world's leading combatives expert, specializing in edged weapons.

Shihan Kevin "KO" Pickron

Kevin "KO" Pickron a co-founder of *"Stick Fit"* is an American Kick boxing Hall of Fame member and one of the sport's true pioneers. The Professional Karate Association (PKA) list Mr. Pickron as one of the world's greatest strikers. In 1992 he won the United States Light-heavy Weight title in the very first tournament ever to allow kick, punch, throw and submission grappling on an organized level. One year before the first UFC and several years before the term MMA would ever be used. As a former member of the United States Sport Jujitsu Team his tenacious fighting style and humble demeanor earned him the reputation internationally as a world class fighter and gentleman. He is the assistant coach for Team USA and currently the chief instructor at BCI Modern Day Warriors located in Hurricane, West Virginia.

Dr. Keith Jeffery

A 30 year Tai Chi veteran is a world leader in the field of Tai Chi for fitness and health promotion. He has created many very popular and effective tai Chi instructional videos and nutritional audio tapes. Much of his time is devoted to teaching 4 Minute Fitness to business and organizations, helping employees learn easy and effective ways to decrease stress and find balance and peace.

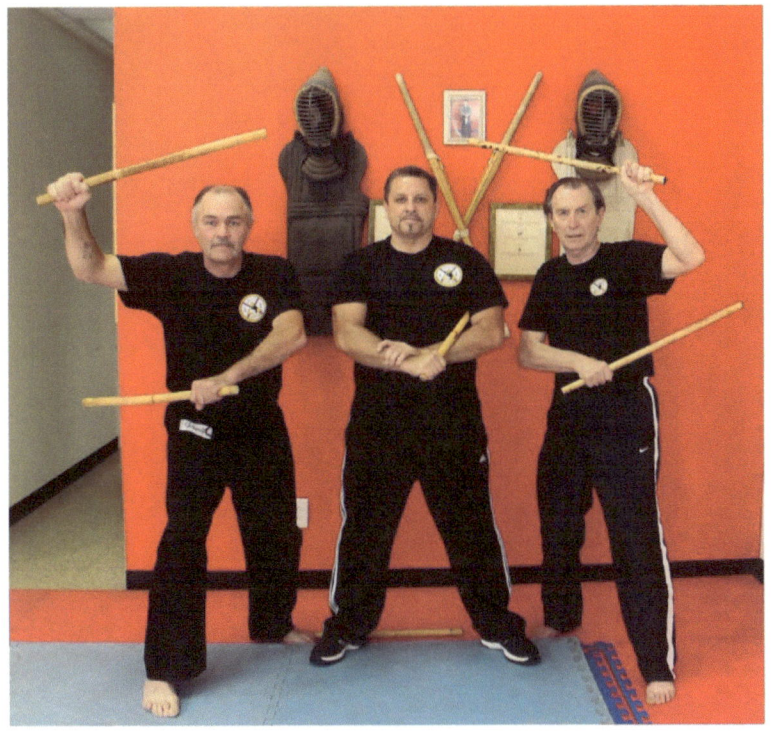

Shihan Kevin "KO" Pickron, Professor Ernie Boggs, and Sensei James Birkle

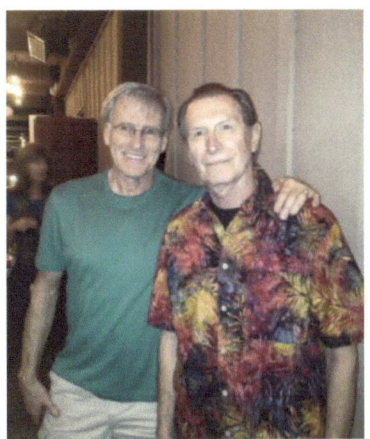

Dr. Keith Jeffery and James Birkle

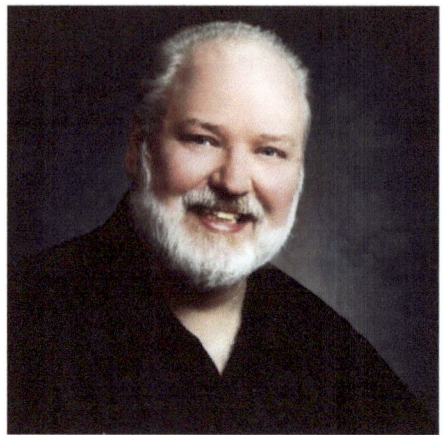

I would also like to thank **Mr. Gary Wittmann** for his assistance and to my family for their undying support of my martial arts training and my first adventure as an author. Without the above mentioned people none of this would have been possible.

-James Birkle

ABOUT THE AUTHOR

Chief Instructor James Birkle

James Birkle, a 73 year old living life by setting the example that age does not mean you can no longer live an active and fulfilling life. Mr. Birkle is a cofounder and the chief instructor for **Stick Fit "Senior Strong."** As a martial artist he holds black belts in two different systems, a 2nd degree black belt in American Kenpo and a 1st degree black belt in Kodenkan Jujitsu. He is also active in Tai Chi and Qiqong and currently continues his martial studies as the oldest student under world renowned martial artist, Professor Ernie Boggs.

Mr. Birkle is a member of the **Independent Martial Arts Federation** and *the **United States Sport Jujitsu Association.*** James Birkle travelled to Geneva, Switzerland in 2013 as part of a team representing the United States. While there he captured the Gold medal in a self defense competition against competitors less than half his age. seniorstickfit.com@gmail.com

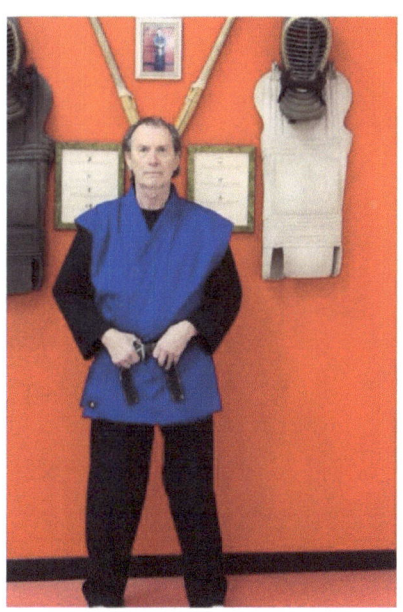

STICK FIT – SENIOR STRONG

This book covers some of the fundamentals of *"Stick Fit - Senior Strong"* as well as basic exercises that are designed to improve the balance, flexibility, breathing and overall fitness of men and women over the age of 65. The exercise routines in this book can be done while standing or sitting making participation possible for everyone. Stick Fit *"Senior Strong"* is a special element of the BCI Stick Fit program that has been designed specifically for men and women who are 65 years of age and older. This 30 minute, easy to learn, low impact, moderately challenging class, was created by world renowned martial artist & fitness instructor, Professor Ernie Boggs with the assistance of martial arts Hall of Fame member, Kevin Pickron and Jim Birkle. Mr. Birkle acts as the President and chief instructor for the *Senior Strong* branch of the BCI Stick Fit program.

Table of Contents

Senior Stick Fit Exercises

Introduction

As people get along in age, the importance of maintaining an active and healthy lifestyle becomes more apparent. Exercise can benefit not only the elderly body, but improve aging minds and moods as well.

Exercise can help combat the effects of aging such as increased feeling of lethargy and moodiness. It can also give you a renewed feeling of self-esteem and independence by boosting your energy and mental awareness. You will find that daily mental stimulation will help you maintain a sharper and more reliable memory.

Likewise, regular exercise can help you manage the most common age-related aches and pains. Regardless of your overall health, it is vital that you start keeping an active lifestyle and boosting your health as early as you can.

Retiring from your work routine does not mean that you should stop being active. Unfortunately, age can prevent many senior citizens from keeping to a set schedule as easily as they once did. They can become tempted to stray from their routine because of the onset of illnesses and other age-related pains, or the inherent fear of sustaining severe injuries from a bad fall. After all, diminished muscle strength and brittle bones means that seniors could already become bedridden simply from losing their balance.

Conversely, they could be genuinely lost when it comes to exercise simply because they had never tried it in their younger years. The reasons they had for excusing themselves from physical activity then, such as boredom or apprehension, could be the same things that are preventing them from starting now.

However, while they might think that being old and frail is a good reason to take it easy, sleeping their days away might actually do them more harm than good. In truth, the key to living a longer and healthier life is regular daily exercise. Nevertheless, they should still be aware of their limitations and realize that they cannot and should not strive to match the stamina and strength of their younger counterparts.

Also, they do not have to worry about needing to actually drag themselves to a gym and engaging in strenuous workouts. There are many exercises that they can easily accomplish and even enjoy doing in the comfort of their own homes.

Whether they are healthy or suffering from small illnesses, they can always find a suitable physical activity that they can incorporate into their daily routine. Stretching in the early mornings or walking around the garden to tend to the flowers can already help your get your blood flowing and keep you energized throughout the day.

Aside from engaging in low impact exercises, it is also important that the elderly keep themselves hydrated at all times. Likewise, they should be more mindful of their breathing and heart rate. Increasing muscle mass will have to take a backseat to simply maintaining muscle strength when it comes to exercise for the elderly.

Deep Breathing Exercises for the Elderly

Breathing exercises are among the easiest and most important physical activities that the elderly should engage in. Proper breathing techniques will strengthen not only their lungs, but promote good heart health and blood circulation as well.

However, when teaching the proper breathing technique, it is vital that you take particular note of how the elderly take in each breath. It is likely that they will hold their breaths in order to help them gain more momentum in exerting physical force. This means that you will have to encourage them to take deeper breaths in order to help them improve their oxygen intake. After all, they will be able to draw more strength from more oxygen rather than from simply holding their breath.

Additionally, it is important that you encourage the elderly to maintain good posture while performing their breathing exercises. The correct posture will help their lungs take in more air regardless of whether they are standing up or sitting down.

Generally, the correct breathing posture requires them to keep their shoulders back and their chests pushed forward. Aside from allowing their lungs to work at their maximum capacity, maintaining this posture will help them become more aware of every single inhale and exhale. As a result, even when they are performing more strenuous exercises, they will be able to give importance to their breathing.

Breathing Exercise while Lying Down

Aside from the lungs, the stomach is one of the main organs that you should focus on during breathing exercises. You should be able to note it expanding and contracting as you inhale and exhale.

While executing breathing exercises while lying down, the first thing you should do is to find a comfortable position. You have the option of bending your knees or placing a pillow underneath your legs if that will make you feel more comfortable. Afterwards, you should place one hand over your chest and the other hand directly underneath your rib cage.

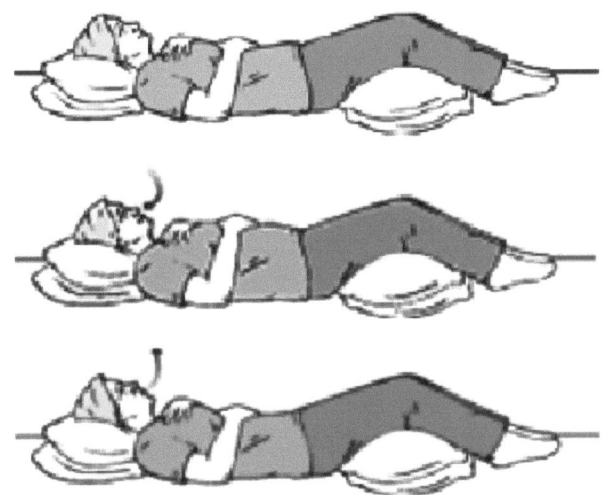

When you take in that first deep breath, you should feel the hand on your chest rise higher than the one on your stomach. If you do not feel your hands moving, that means that your breathing is too shallow. You should therefore remember to be more conscious of your next intake of air and breath deeper.

After executing the proper inhale, you must then focus on the correct exhaling technique. While keeping your hand on your stomach, you should feel your stomach as your ribs fall after each exhale. Use your stomach muscles to help you prolong each exhale for a minimum of 5 seconds at a time. Maximizing your lung capacity will help you breathe easier as well as make you more mindful of each breath.

Seated Breathing Exercise

Some elderly might have problems with getting up from a lying position. In this case, they might find it easier to execute breathing exercises while sitting down.

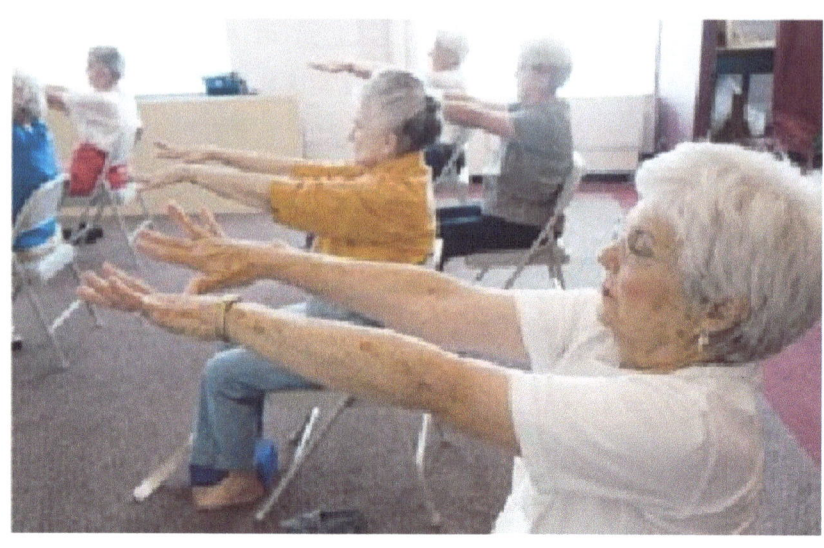

After finding a stable chair to sit on, you will need to let your hands Rest loosely at your sides. Then you should take a deep breath and feel your chest rise while keeping your shoulders back. As you exhale, slowly extend your arms forward and start humming single note.

You will undoubtedly feel tired as you extend the note so you will have to draw strength from your stomach muscles. Prolong the note for as long as you can and slowly lower your arms when you feel ready to take the next breath. This exercise will help strengthen your stomach muscles as well as help increase the amount of oxygen in your bloodstream.

Perform these exercises with a minimum of ten repetitions. Each repetition is composed of one deep inhale and exhale. Additionally, it is recommended that you perform these breathing exercises outdoors if possible in order to get some fresh air into your system.

Balance Exercises for the Elderly

Exercises that focus on balance and overall mobility are of particular importance for the elderly. They will have to pay more attention to maintaining their center of gravity whether they are simply sitting down or walking around. Although you may not realize it, constantly shifting your position or bending down already requires you to engage your body in a number of different ways.

Unfortunately, aging can take its toll on both your muscles and your bones. This means that a bad fall could already cause a serious injury in an elderly individual. Therefore, seniors as well as their family members should take the necessary precautions in order to ensure their safety even while at home.

The ankles are some of the body parts that play the biggest role in maintaining good balance. Strengthening your ankles will help strengthen your awareness of your center of gravity. As a result, you will find it easier to balance while keeping your good posture.

However, before you engage in any type of balancing exercise, it is recommended that you consult with your doctor or tending physician. It is vital that he gives his consent especially if you have not been particularly active for a long time.

Preparing for Balancing Exercises

After you have acquired your doctor's necessary approval, you can then establish an exercise routine that will help you improve your balance. The first thing that you should do before doing any form of exercise is to properly warm up your muscles and joints.

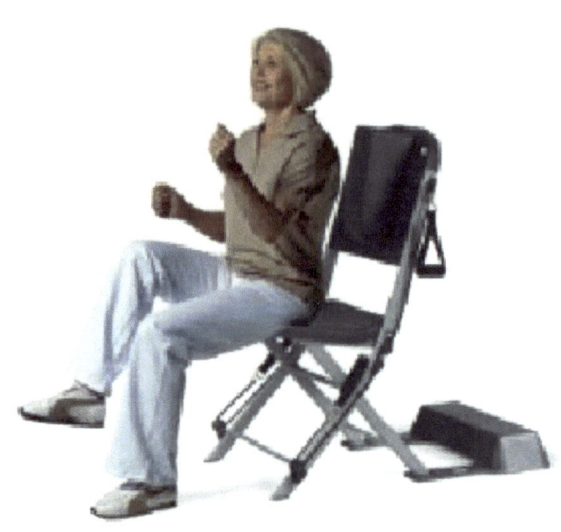

One easy warm-up that you can perform in a seated or standing position is simply marching in place. While keeping your back straight, alternately lift each foot from the ground. Repeat the procedure for three to five minutes in order to get your blood pumping and raise your body temperature.

If you feel that you will not easily lose your balance, you can also create large circles using your arms while you march in place. After a few rounds, your muscles should be ready to perform more strenuous movements.

Since your main goal will be to strengthen your ankles, you will also have to make sure that those ankle joints are sufficiently warmed-up. If you performed the first warm-up while seated, you will have to stand up for this next exercise and stand behind your chair. Hold on to the backrest of the chair for support and lift one leg off the ground. Slowly rotate the foot in a clockwise motion for ten counts. Afterwards, slowly rotate it in a counter clockwise

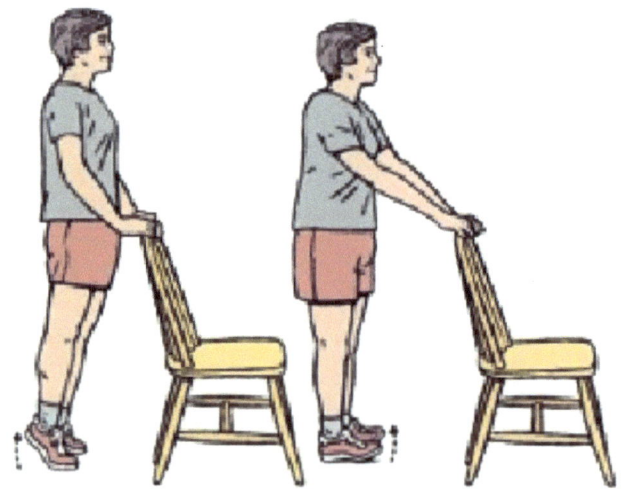

motion for another ten counts. Repeat the process on your other foot.

Standing Balance Exercise

Standing on one leg is one of the most common balancing exercises that you can easily practice at home. However, in order to prevent any accidental falls, it is best if you have a strong solid surface or sturdy chair that you can hold onto.

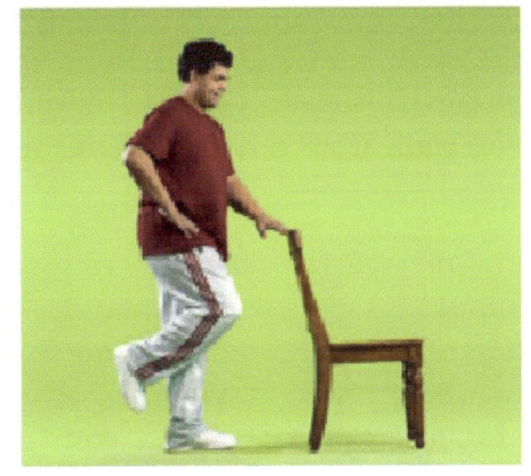

Next, you should lightly grasp the chair from behind and slowly raise your right foot toward your left knee. Hold this position for ten counts before you lower your foot. Do the same thing with your left leg. Repeat the process until each leg has accomplished 3 to 5 repetitions.

Challenge yourself by crossing your arms over your chest while keeping the chair within easy reach as you stand on one leg. Similarly, you can try closing your eyes or rotating your foot while keeping one leg raised.

Repeating this simple exercise will already help strengthen your ankles and hips. Both body parts are essential in helping you improve your stability.

Walking Exercises for Balance

For an even more challenging exercise routine, you will have to let go of the chair and start walking around. Walking may seem like a simple activity, but in this case you will have to pay particular attention to your balance as you walk from one end of the room to the other.

The first thing you should do is to stand adjacent to one wall in order to help you walk in a straight line. As you makeyour way forward, you will have to double-check that the heel of your leading foot will directly touch the toes of the other.

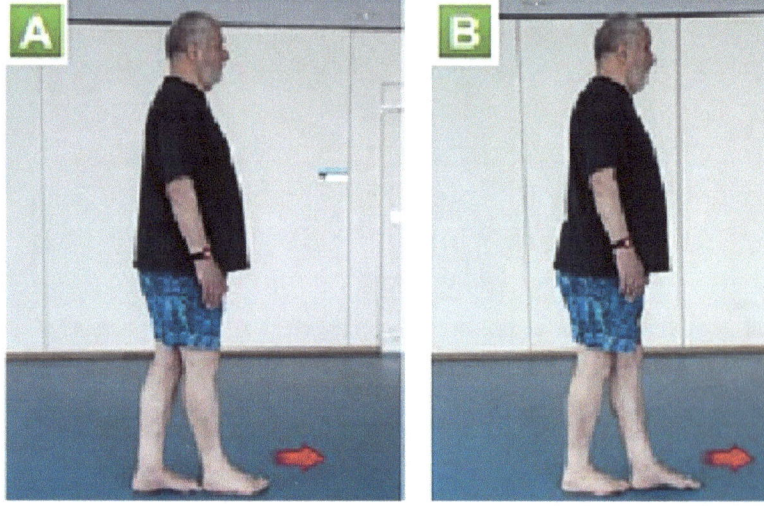

Remember to keep your back straight as you continue walking heel to toe. If you are having trouble with keeping your balance, you can lightly touch the adjacent wall for support.

Once you reach the other side of the room, you can choose to increase the difficulty of the exercise according to your preference. One good challenge is to walk backwards while maintaining the heel to toe stance.

However, as with any exercise, always make sure that you have competently performed the most basic steps before incorporating any extra movements or challenges. You should make sure that you are mentally and physically prepared before you make any type of progression. Likewise, make sure that you take a break and sit down during any instance that you feel dizzy or out of breath.

Ways to Relieve and Manage Stress for Senior Health

Although retirement will provide you with an overall sense of peace, it does not guarantee that you will not be susceptible to other potential stressors. Other factors such as volatile relationships and unstable finances could be a source of stress for many seniors.

Unfortunately, for those who are getting on in age, these stressors do not only diminish your peace of mind, but adversely affect your health as well. Highly stressful situations could cause spikes in blood pressure or even cause heart attacks.

Therefore, it is important that you find ways to manage your stress even during your elderly years. In order to help you maintain your health, you can simply take note of a few effective stress management methods.

Meditation Techniques

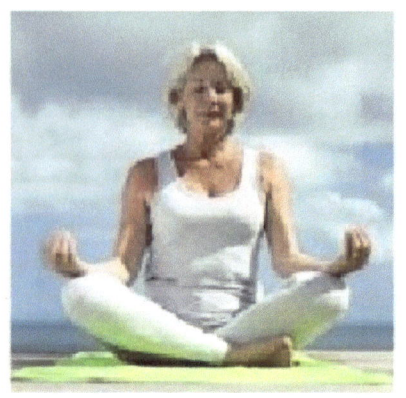

Regularly practicing meditation techniques will not only help you deal with current stressors. It will also prevent you from succumbing to any future stressful situations. Even if everyone else around you is in a state of panic, you will still be able to stay alert and composed.

Additionally, meditation is an activity that you can easily perform without the use of any additional equipment. You simply need to find a quiet space and find your center in order to experience relief from stress.

Although there are many different ways to meditate, the two main meditation techniques are concentrative and non-concentrative. Concentrative techniques require you to focus on an external object while you attempt to clear your mind. The objects can appeal to your sense of sight, such as a candle flame, or to your sense of hearing, such as a song or mantra.

Conversely, non-concentrative meditation techniques require you to look inward and become more mindful of your own body. You will need to pay close attention to your breathing while noting the different sounds in your environment.

Regardless of the technique you choose, you will undoubtedly reap the many benefits of daily meditation. Likewise, depending on your specific needs or preferences, you can even devise a meditation routine that combines both techniques.

Yoga

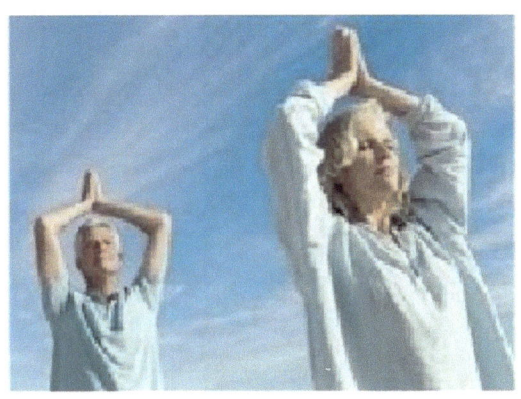

Similar to meditation, yoga is another activity that can help you reduce your stress levels and promote overall well-being. Additionally, yoga is a low-impact exercise that can help you increase your flexibility. Likewise, it can improve your strength and endurance.

Regardless of your faith or fitness level, you can find a yoga style that will help you de-stress. In addition, you need not be pressured about keeping to strict routine when practicing yoga. Unlike other exercises, you can perform this activity on an either daily or weekly basis without incurring any adverse effects.

Tai Chi

Another low impact form of exercise that is similar to yoga is Tai Chi. However, unlike yoga which can be practiced at any time during the day, Tai Chi is more often **practiced** during early mornings.

Practitioners prefer to exercise outside to take advantage of the cool morning air for a more comfortable environment. Unfortunately, this means that seniors might have a harder time finding a Tai Chi buddy or group since they must bewilling to wake up early for every session.

Never the less, waking up early will undoubtedly prove beneficial for those willing to make the sacrifice. Regularly practicing the slow and controlled Tai Chi move and stances will not only help you lessen your stress, but improve your balance as well.

Water Aerobics

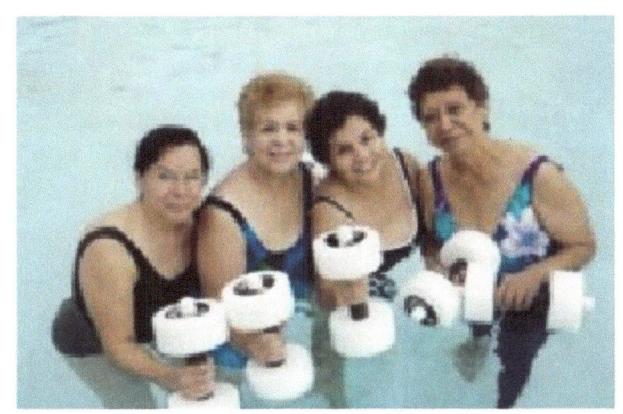

Sometimes you might want a change of environment while you de-stress. In such cases, you can opt to engage in stress reducing exercises that you can perform while floating in pool.

Water aerobics is a form of exercise that not only lessens the stress on your mind, but decreases the stress on your joints and muscles as well. The water will enable you to easily use weights that you would not be able to hold while on land. This means that you will be able to increase your muscle strength while still maintaining a relaxed state of mind.

Ultimately, the stress relieving method that you choose for yourself should be one that you actually enjoy doing. You will find it easier to ease that method into your daily routine if it is something that you find enjoyable. Whether you choose to practice yoga or tai chi or any other method, they will undoubtedly help you keep your cool even during the most turbulent times of your senior years.

Building Self Confidence in the Elderly

As people grow older, they find that their bodies can change in many surprising ways. Unfortunately for the elderly, they might find that those changes can be negative at most. They will be unable to do many of the things that they used to take for granted such as running or eating anything they wanted. Likewise, they will find it difficult to do simple tasks such as reading, listening, or even speaking without exerting effort.

All of these limitations can exact a toll on the egos of seniors and diminish their self-esteem. The elderly can end up feeling useless and start retreating into themselves while simply waiting for death.

Fortunately, there are simple steps that can be taken to help the elderly regain their self-confidence. However, these steps are not meant to be performed alone. You will require the assistance of your loved ones in order to help you find your sense of purpose and thirst for life once again. Although these steps will not reverse the toll that aging has taken on your body, these will at least help you achieve a more positive state of mind.

.

Look at the Bright Side

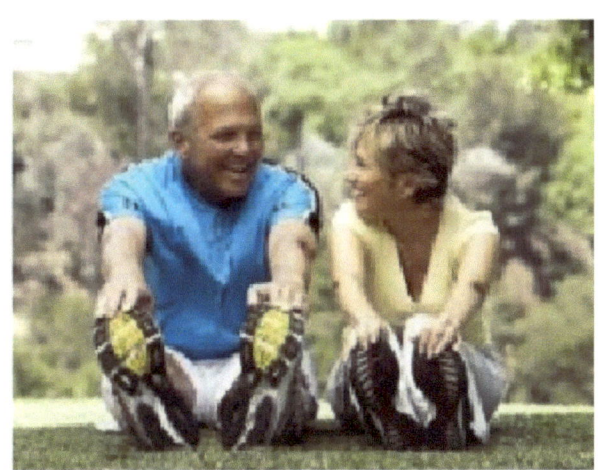

One of the most difficult aspects of aging is watching your friends and loved ones leave this life one by one. Although these events alone can already cause much distress, knowing that you could be next only adds to the anxiety.

For this reason, it is important that you learn to focus on the present instead of imagining all of the bleak future possibilities. Even if you can no longer enjoy all of your past hobbies, you can still find ways to keep both your mind and your body active.

Although you might not be able to jog or run anymore, you can still engage in brisk walking or swimming. Likewise, if you find your eyesight fading, you can choose to listen to audio books or to soothing music instead. By finding a new way of doing things, you will be able to keep doing what you love even as you get older.

Engage in Regular Physical Activity

Exercise will help improve your strength and physical appearance as well as give you a much needed endorphin boost. Additionally, seeing the immediate changes that regular physical activities have on your body will help you feel more confident. Aside from the physical benefits, exercise can also improve their emotional well-being. By performing 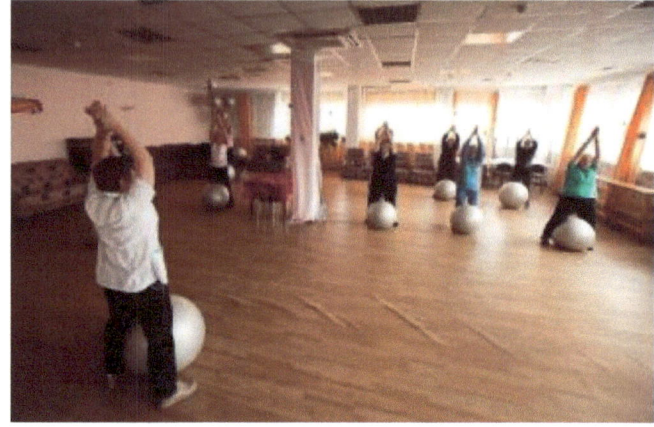 the exercise routines with a group or with a loved one, the elderly will be able to feel more secure in their ability to make new friends or to strengthen old bonds.

Share those Stories

The elderly can often feel alienated from the younger generations due to their different sets of values and experiences. However, those experiences can often hold invaluable insights that only they can share to their descendants.

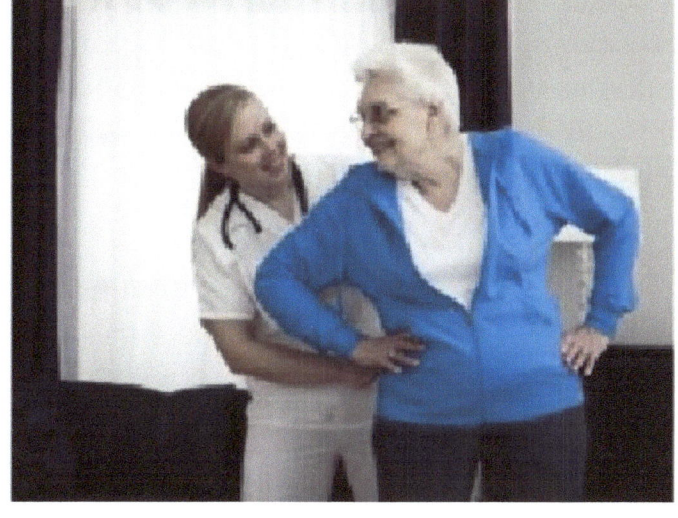

Therefore, you should be proud of the many experiences that have made you into who you are today. You could have been an avid traveler in the past or a survivor of a great event and those are things that you should not keep to yourself.

Share them with anyone who is willing to lend an ear or be more proactive and share your stories to the young schoolchildren who have only ever read about such things in history books. In this way, you will be able to build your self-confidence while finding a way to contribute to your community. In the end, you simply need to find a more positive and alternative way of looking at your life in order to regain self-confidence in your older years. Although your body might not be as strong as it once was, that should not prevent you from doing what you want and continuing to make a difference.

Being Active through Results

Oftentimes, the increasing amount of age-related aches and illnesses you experience enables you to make more excuses to avoid engaging in physical activities. Although you are aware of the benefits that exercise can give you, you could still have a problem with keeping yourself motivated with the passage of time.

In such cases, aside from finding the right exercise routine, you should also focus on attaining and keeping your motivation. After all, once you are able to consistently practice your exercises, you will be able to achieve results much faster.

Set Realistic Goals

Seeing immediate positive results is one of the easiest ways to motivate yourself to stick to your routine. Although you should have a long-term goal, you should set daily goals as well. In this way, you will feel as though you are achieving something every day. After all, the elderly would much rather focus on the present rather than constantly worry about the things that could happen in the future.

Additionally, you can also track your daily progress to give you a more concrete way of measuring your achievements. After all, some changes could be unnoticeable at first glance. However, if you have a written point of comparison regarding those changes, you will be able to better appreciate the effects of your exercise routine.

One example would be balancing on one leg for 10 counts one day and balancing for 15 counts the next. Although you will not notice any immediate physical effects, that measurable progress will prove that you are growing stronger every day.

Work with a Partner or Group

Aside from making your exercise routine safer and more enjoyable, a workout buddy will be able to provide you with immediate feedback. However, you should ensure that you can trust this person or persons to actually give you honest feedback without sugar coating your capabilities.

Additionally, these workout buddies will be able to give you that much needed push and support to keep going. They will also be able to identify your short comings and help you overcome them. Once you have overcome those obstacles, they will then be able to give constructive criticism that will motivate you to try more challenging moves.

In a similar way, you can also choose to use electronic gadgets such as heart monitors or pedometers to supply direct and objective feedback. These gadgets will let you know whether you are achieving your daily physical quota. Likewise, you will be able to find more fun in your otherwise repetitive routine by treating those numerical results as a challenging game.

Take Things One at a Time

If you are unable to accomplish a daily goal, you should not let that minor setback determine the tone of your entire week. Be more flexible in your routine take everything in stride. After all, your physical activities are for your own benefit and one less day will not really have a big impact on your overall well-being and progress.

In the end, the key to finding and keeping your motivation is to take things one step at a time. Consistency, much like exercise results, is not something that you can achieve overnight. Therefore, you should make it a point to find daily enjoyment in your routine in order to help you stay motivated week after week.

WARM-UP EXERCISES

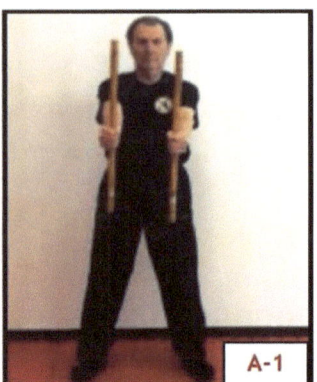 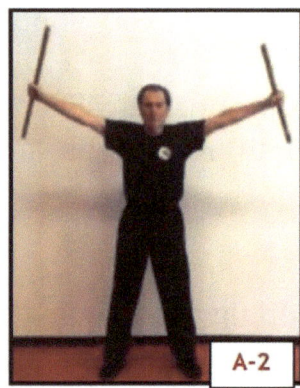 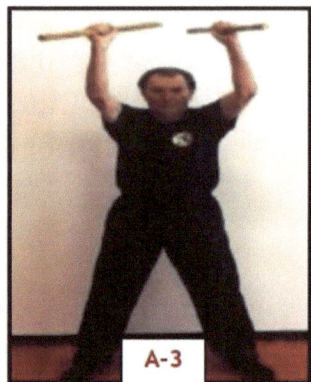 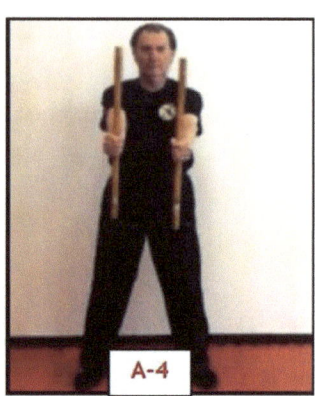

STICK ROTATIONS
Start with feet shoulder distance apart and sticks held directly in front of your body, while twisting your wrist back and forth, simultaneously spread your arms open wide, then lift above the head and back down in front to the starting position. (Photos A-1 thru A-4)

STRETCHING WITH THE STICKS
Start with feet shoulder distance apart and one stick held with both hands directly above your head as seen below in Photo B-1, take a deep breath, then slowly turn to the left, keeping your back straight while exhaling to full range of motion. Return to starting position and take another deep breath, then repeat the movement by slowly turning to the right as you exhale to the full range of motion as seen in photos B-2 thru B-4. Then from the starting position slowly lean left while breathing out, return to start position and repeat the stretch to the right as seen in photos B-5 thru B-8. Now from the starting position take a deep breath and slowly lean forward keeping your head up and arms fully extended as you slowly exhale to your full range of motion, stretching your lower back and hamstring muscles as seen in photos B-9 thru B-12.

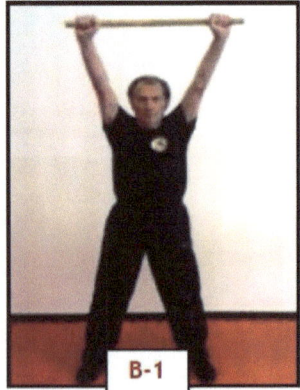 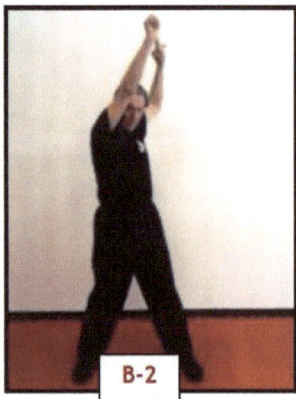 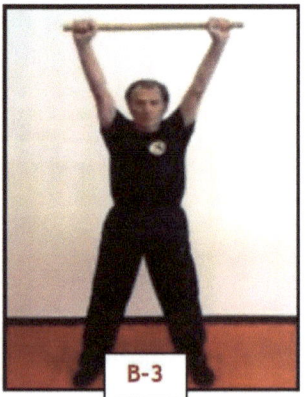 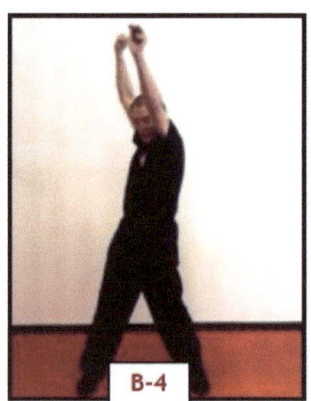

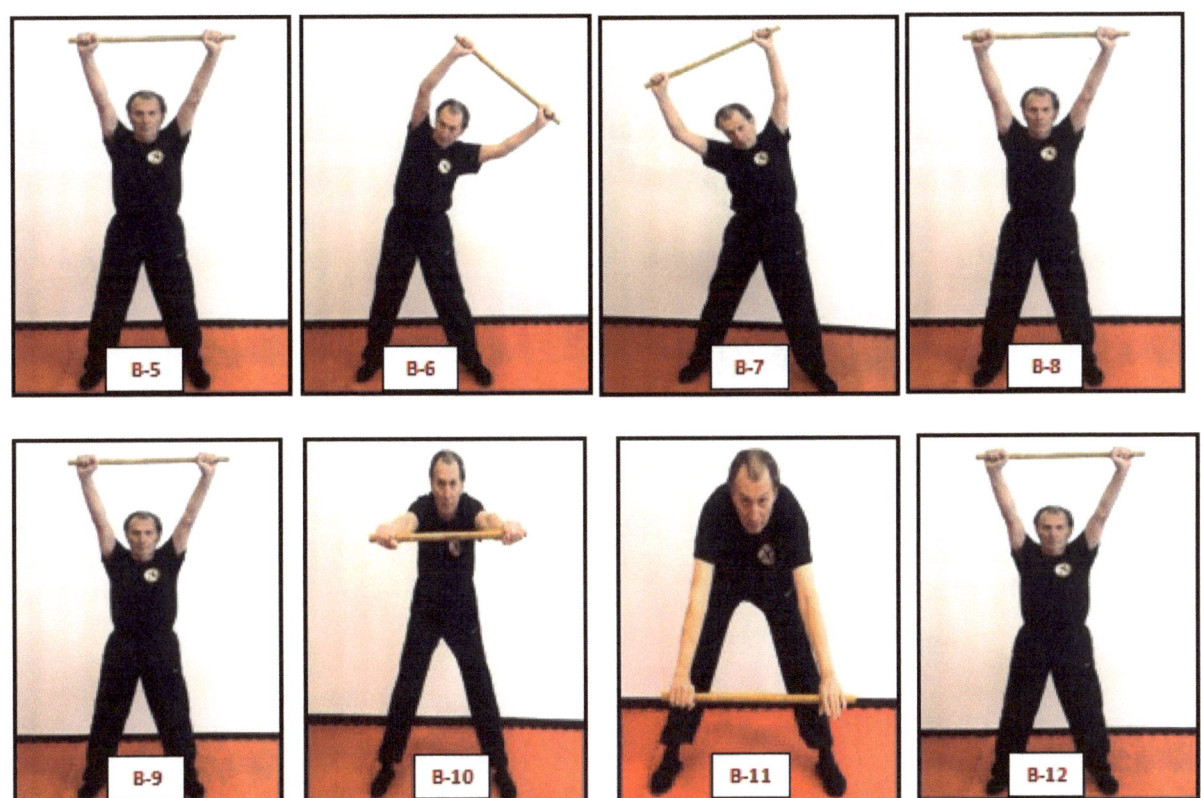

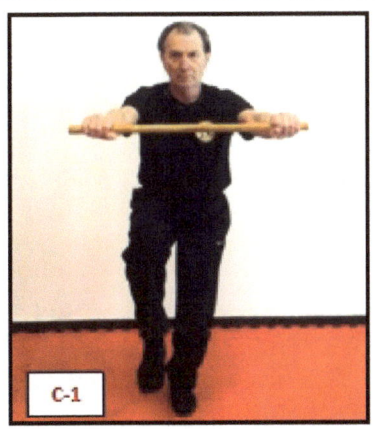

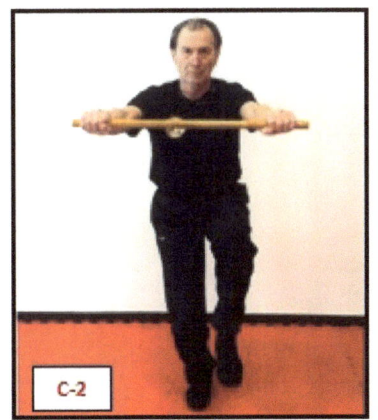

BALANCE EXERCISE

Holding the stick with both hands directly out in front of your chest take a breath in. Then as you exhale raise your right leg slowly and hold for a count of 3 then slowly lower the foot to the floor. Repeat with other leg as seen in Photos C-1 and C-2.

Stick Drills and the Commodity to Self Defense

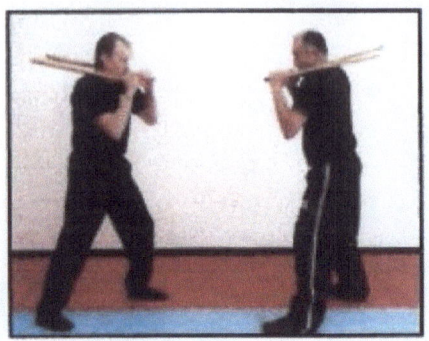

Starting position for all standing.

The Two Count or Cob-Cob

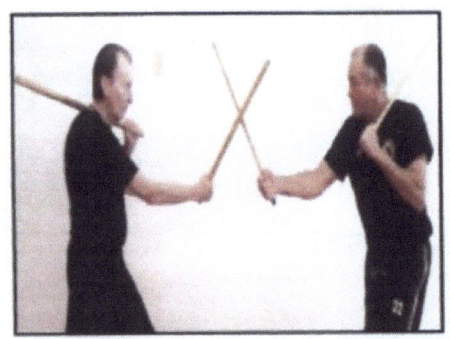 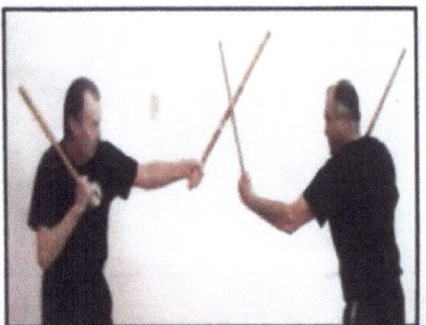

FIRST MOVEMENT; the sticks meet high while executing an *Angle One* with the right hand, then immediately repeat the same movement with the left hand. Repeating the pattern with as many repetitions as desired - left right - left right or One Two - One Two thus the name Two Count.

FROM A SEATED POSITION

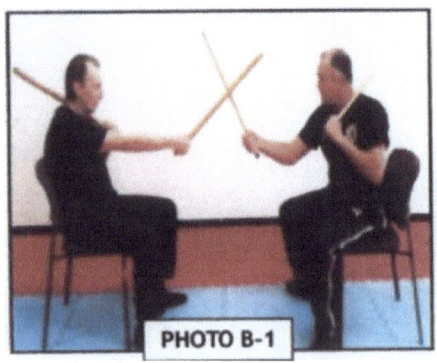 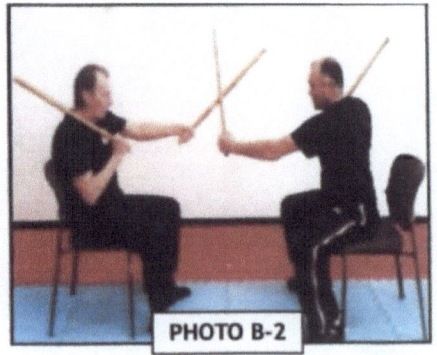

FIVE BASIC ANGLES OF ATTACK AND DEFENSE

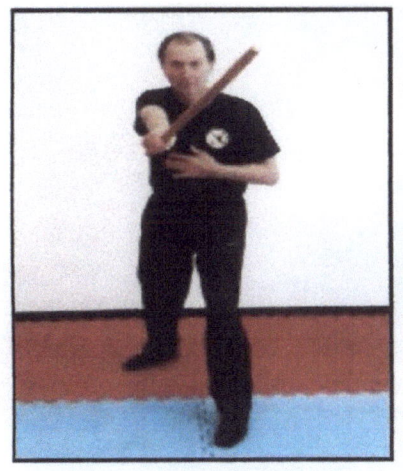

ANGLE ONE
A downward diagonal slash, stab, or strike toward the left side of the defender's head, neck, or torso.

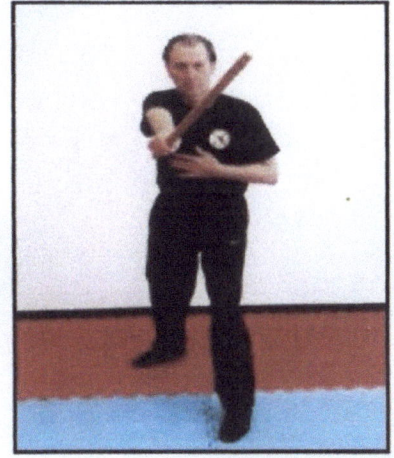

ANGLE TWO
A downward diagonal slash, stab, or strike toward the right side of the defender's head, neck, or torso.

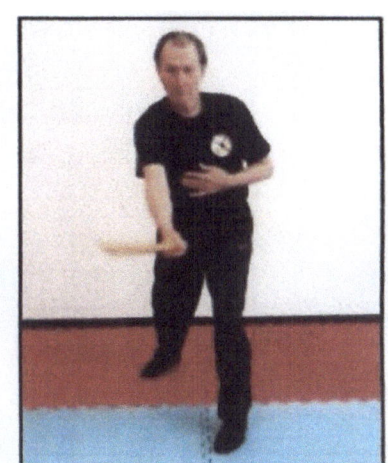

ANGLE THREE
A horizontal attack to the left side of the defender's torso in the ribs, side, or hip region

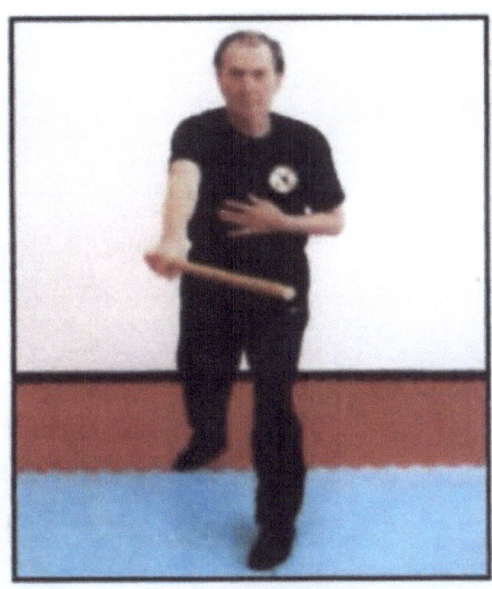

ANGLE FOUR
A horizontal attack to the right side of the defender's torso in the ribs, side, or hip region.

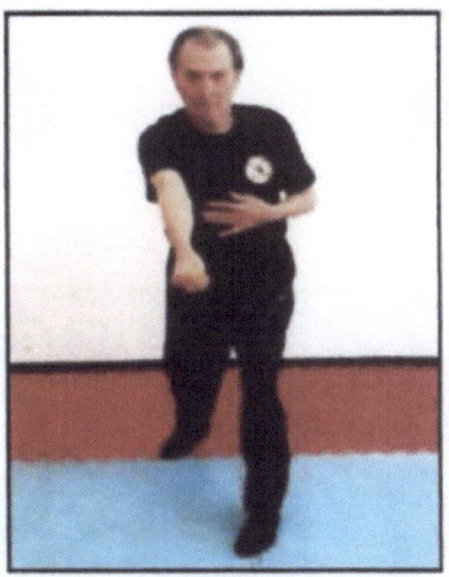

ANGLE FIVE
A jabbing, lunging, or punching attack directed straight toward the defender's center front.

The Three Count

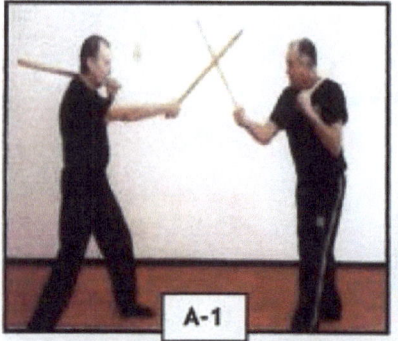 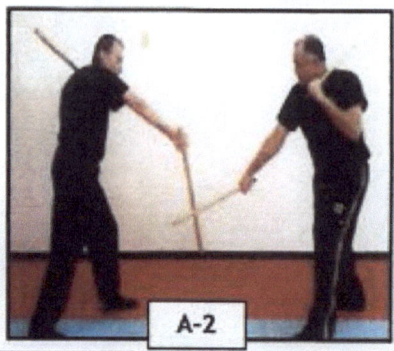 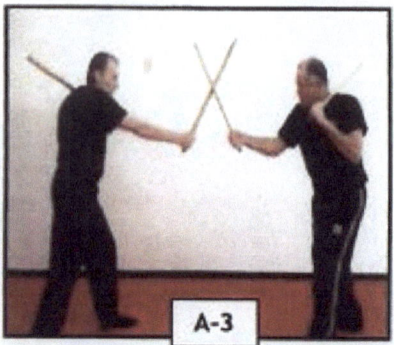

FIRST MOVEMENT; the sticks meet high while executing an *Angle One* and following on through until the sticks meet again low in a downward blocking position...then immediately bring the stick back up until they meet once again in a backhand position as in the *Angle Two* strike. Photos A-1 thru A-3

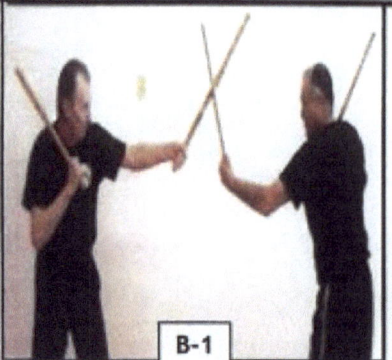 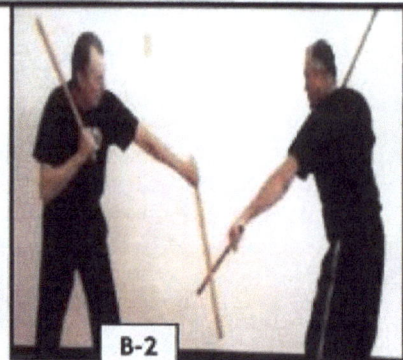 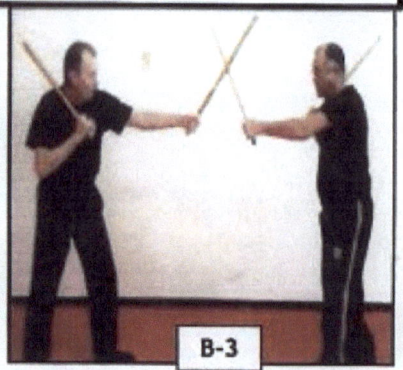

Then repeat the same pattern with the left hand (Photos B1 - B2 & B3) and continue with as many repetitions
as you want. It is referred to as the *three-count* because the sticks meet three times in each exchange. This

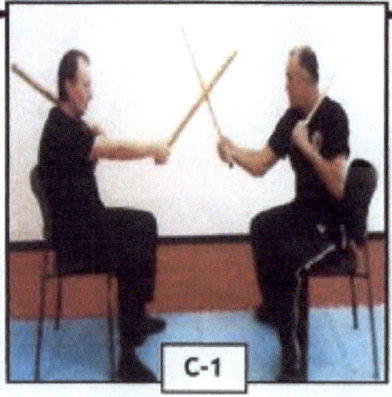 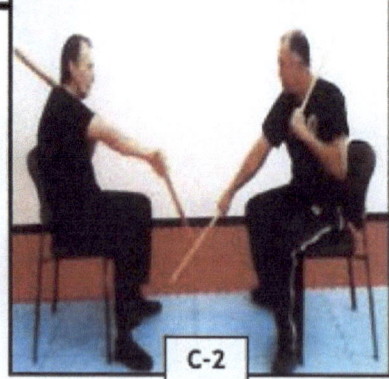 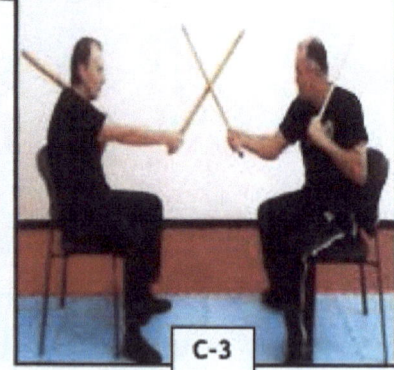

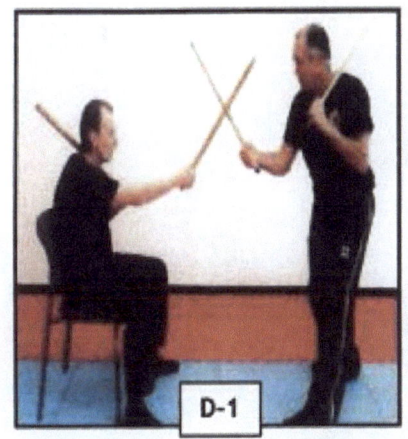 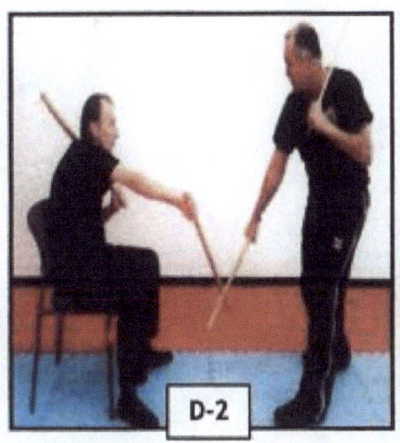 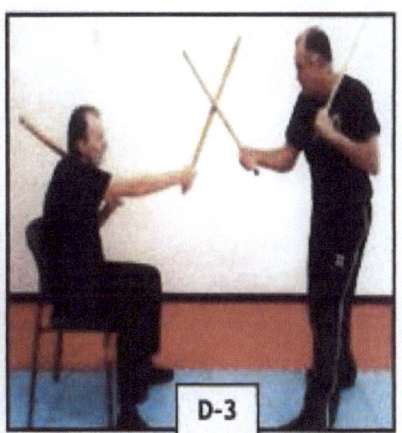

Three Count Exercise Without Sticks

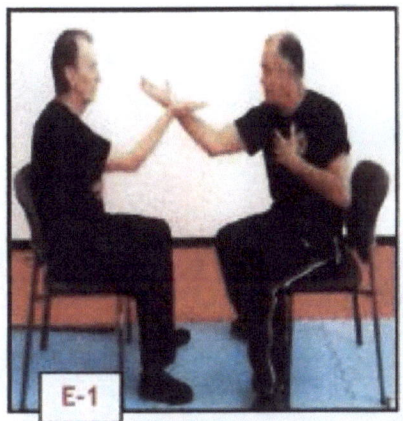 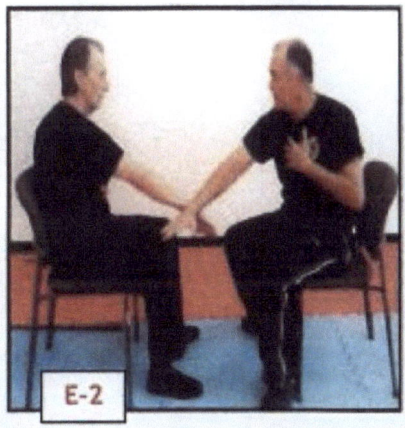 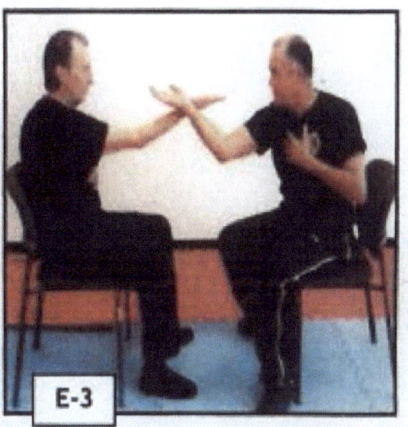

The "Three Count" drill can be done without sticks and serve as a sensitivity, focus and relaxation exercise.
(Photos E1 thru E3). Below in a empty hand self defense situation. Aggressor grabs the wrist, Mr. Birkle uses the three count movement pushing out & downward then immediately snapping back up to

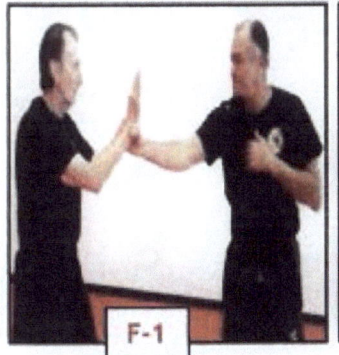 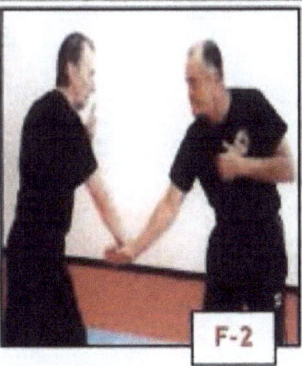 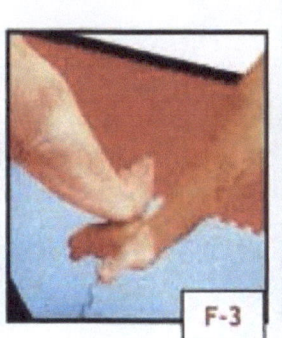 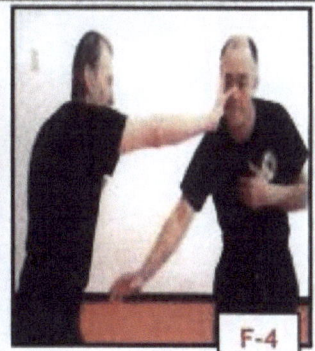

Three Count Exercise Without Sticks

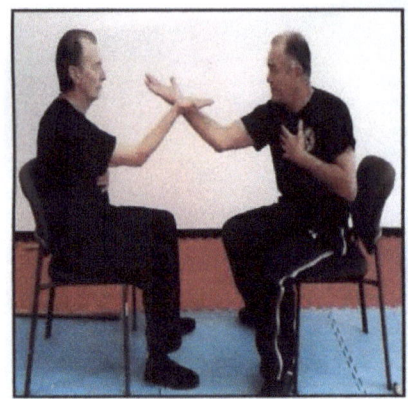 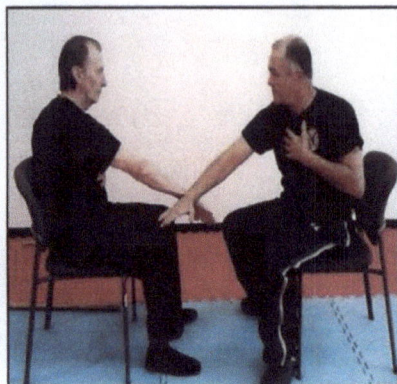 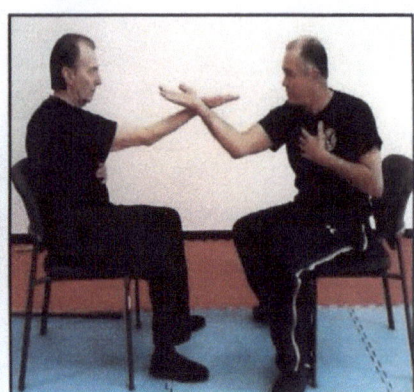

Self Defense Applications

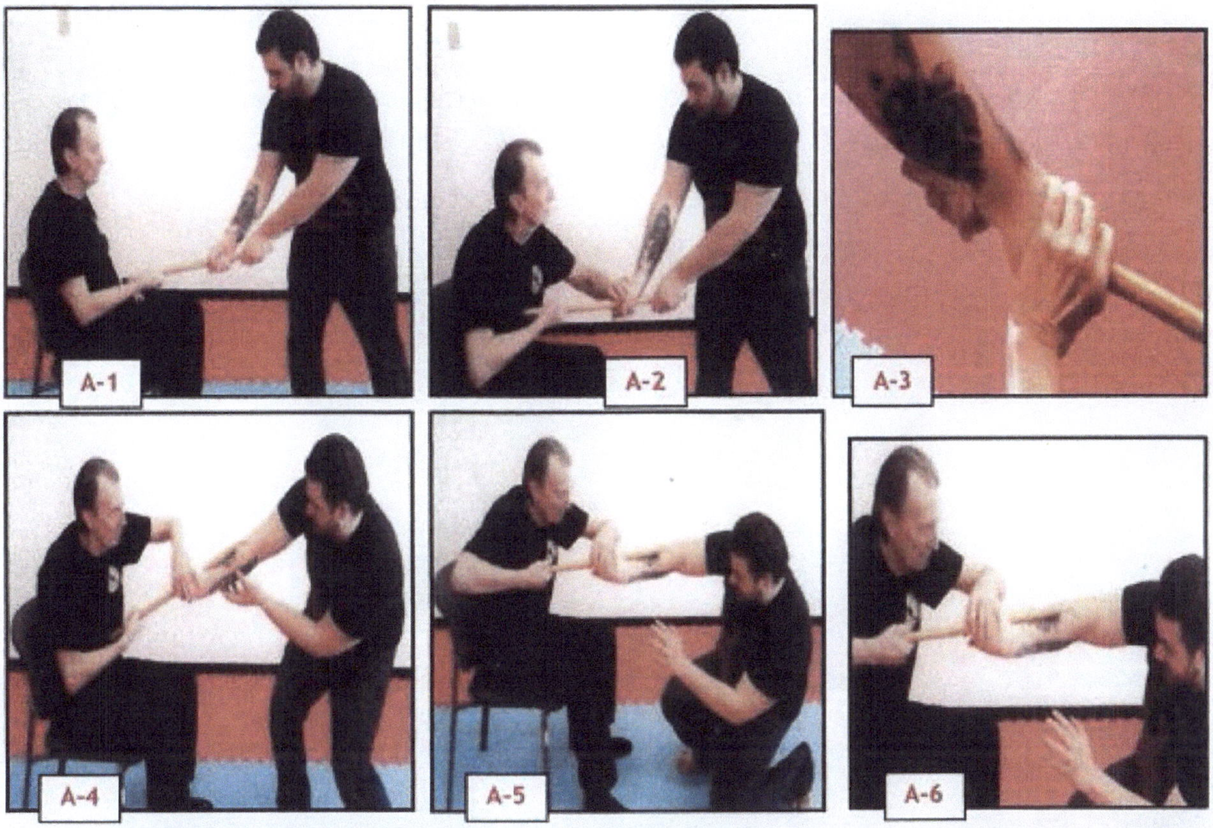

An aggressor tries to take the stick away; while maintaining a grip with his right hand (Photo A-1), Mr. Birkle uses his left hand to trap the aggressor's lead hand (Photos A-2 & A-3), then using leverage he rolls the stick to the outside of the aggressor's wrist and rest on top (Photo A-4), finishing by lifting the rear of the stick he brings the aggressor down with a painful wrist lock (Photo A-5 & A-6). The same technique can be applied from a standing position just follow the same steps as before (Photos B-1 thru B-3)

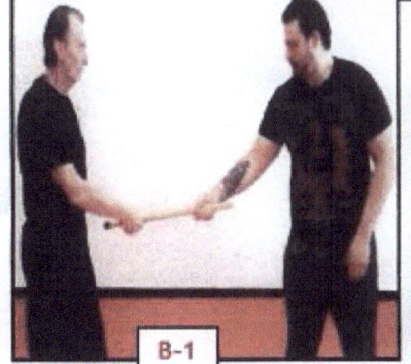
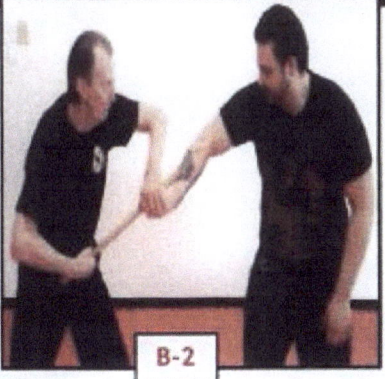
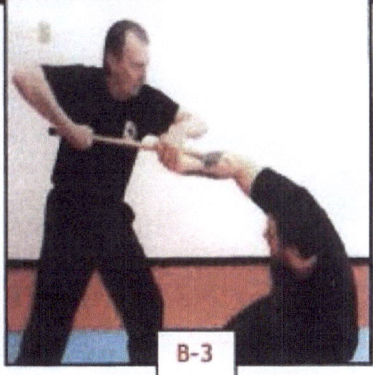

Self Defense Without The Stick

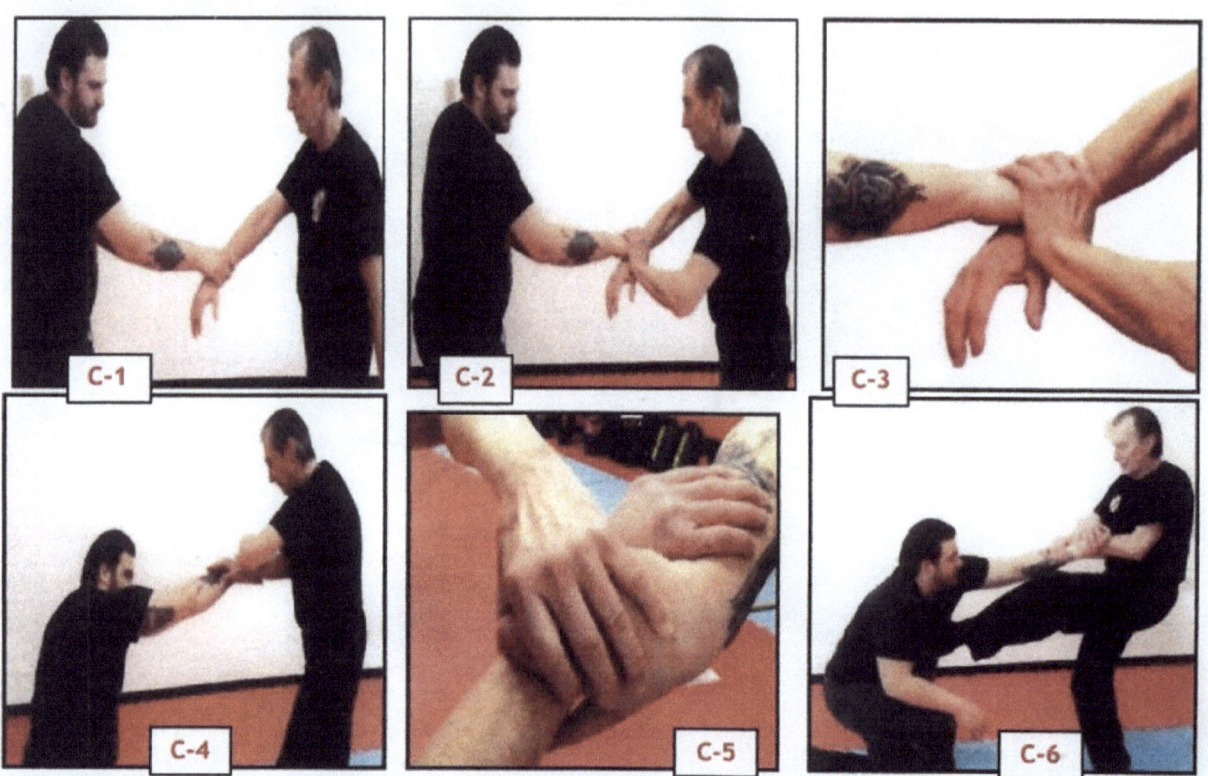

This same defensive technique will work without a stick as well. The aggressor uses a cross-body grab on Mr. Birkle's right wrist with his right hand (Photo C-1), following the same procedures as before, Mr. Birkle traps the aggressor's fingers so he cannot release his grip (Photos C-2 & C-3), then rolls his own hand to the outside of the aggressor's wrist while maintaining a trap on the aggressor's fingers, he presses in a circular motion towards the ground with right hand forcing the aggressor down. He then follows up with a front kick to the aggressor's neck (Photos C-4, C-5 and C-6).

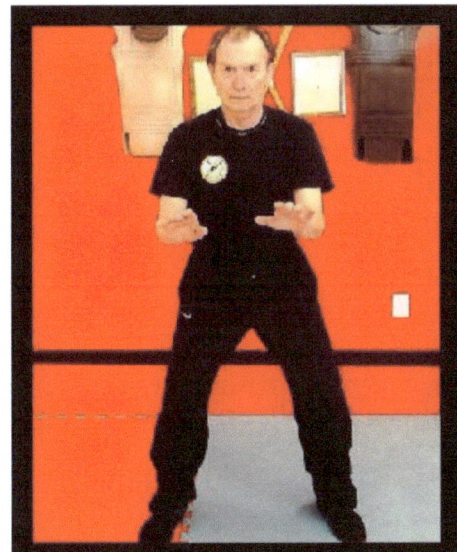 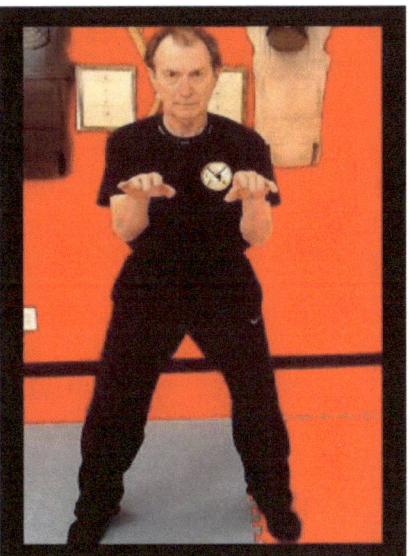

"Let peace and serinty be with you as you workout everyday."

–Sensei James Birkle

In Conclusion

You should never let old age cause you to succumb to a sedentary lifestyle. It is vital that you engage in regular physical activity in order to maintain your well-being and senior health.

However, you should still ensure that you obtain the consent of your attending physician before you start any form of exercise routine. Your body is not a strong or flexible as it once was. Therefore, your doctor will be better able to assess your physical condition and recommend the appropriate exercises for your age and fitness level.

Likewise, he will be able to inform you regarding the possible effects your exercises could have on any form of medication that you could be taking. After all, growing old often comes with various medicines that you will have to ingest just to help you deal with or control any age-related aches and illnesses.

Aside from the actual exercise routine, the elderly should also take particular note of their warm-up stretches and exercises. You should make sure that you start slowly and only move onto more challenging movements once all of your joints and muscles have been sufficiently warmed-up. Take your time and allot at least five minutes for stretching exercises and five more minutes for light cardio exercises before you move on to your actual routine.

Finally, due to the particular importance of maintaining health in late adulthood, you should ensure that you choose a physical activity that you can sustain for a prolonged period. You will find it easier to stick to a routine if you actually find an activity enjoyable to accomplish.

Likewise, if a physical activity causes you to feel dizzy or short of breath, simply find another more suitable activity. You should remember to be mindful of your body and not stress yourself out too much. Exercise should not cause you to lose your self-confidence by highlighting your shortcomings. Instead, it should be a means to increase your endurance, flexibility, balance, and overall happiness.